MW01537040

10 Steps to have happy teeth

Dental Prevention

Written and Illustrated
by Tamara Arauz
A.K.A
Happimola

©2018 Tamara Arauz
All rights reserved.

To my parents and husband.
They motivate me to follow my dreams.

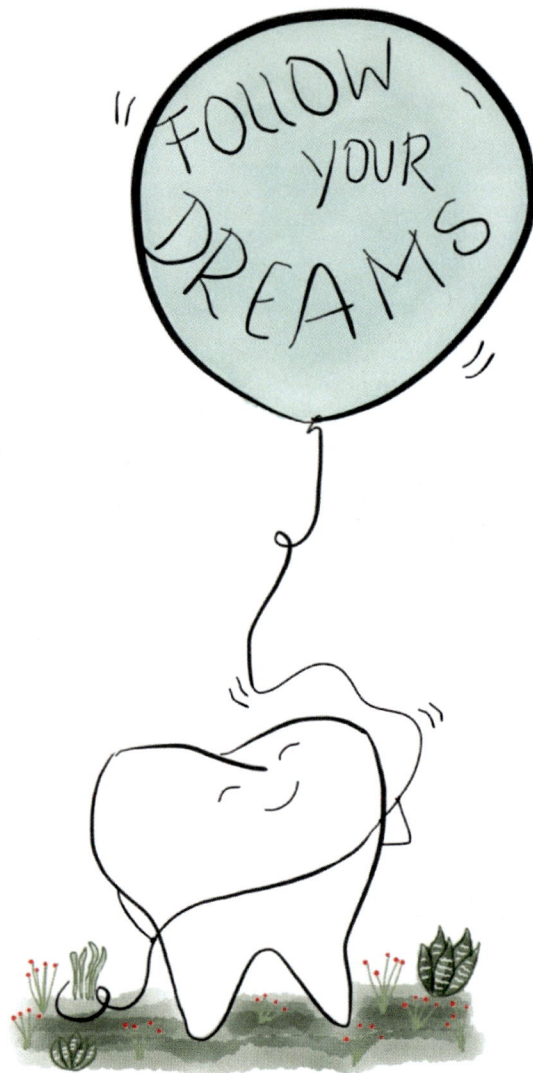

In this guide I explain 10 steps to achieve healthy and happy teeth!

Why happy teeth?

Well, because if you are happy, you feel more motivated to do fun stuff like playing, reading a book, jumping around, doing school projects, and studying.

With this book I want you to feel the same motivation and happiness on taking care of your teeth. If you are happy your teeth will be happy too! Start having good habits!!
A very important one is brushing your teeth every day.

Enjoy the drawings, and I hope you like the surprises at the end of the book! At the end of each page, you'll find a square to draw or take notes on! Happy reading!

Draw here

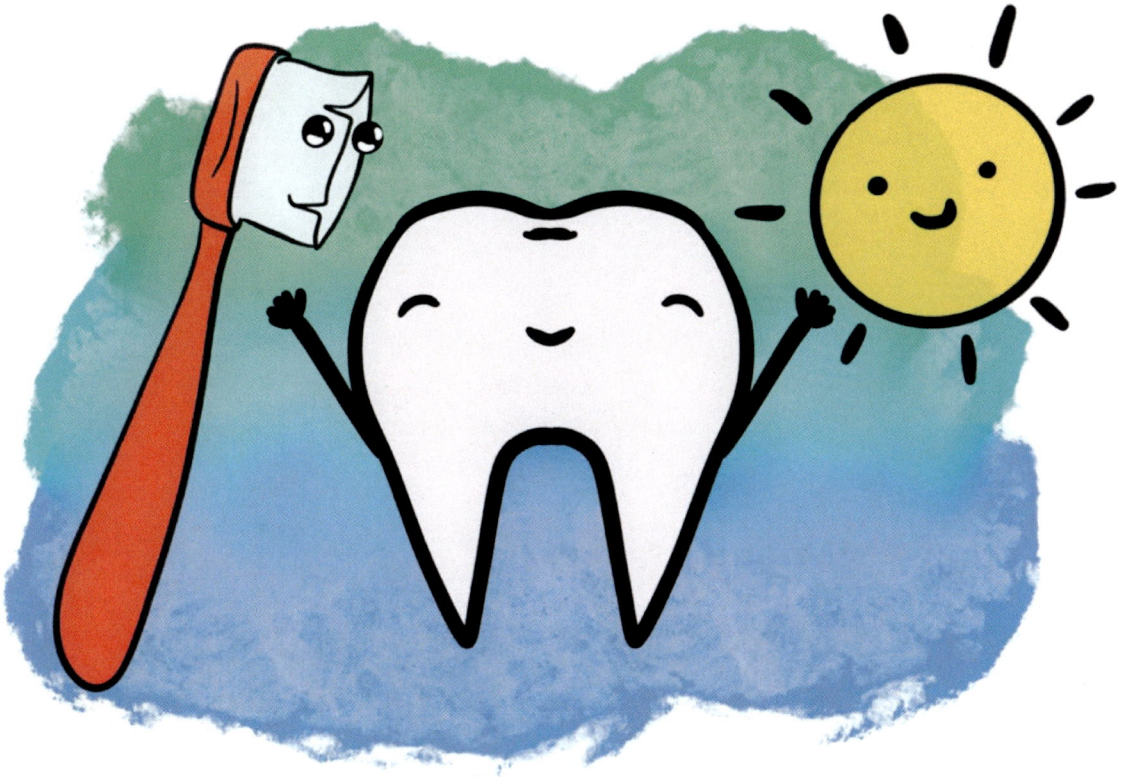

Draw here

BABY TEETH

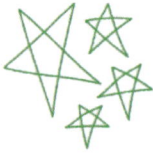
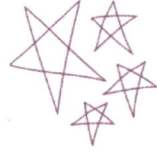

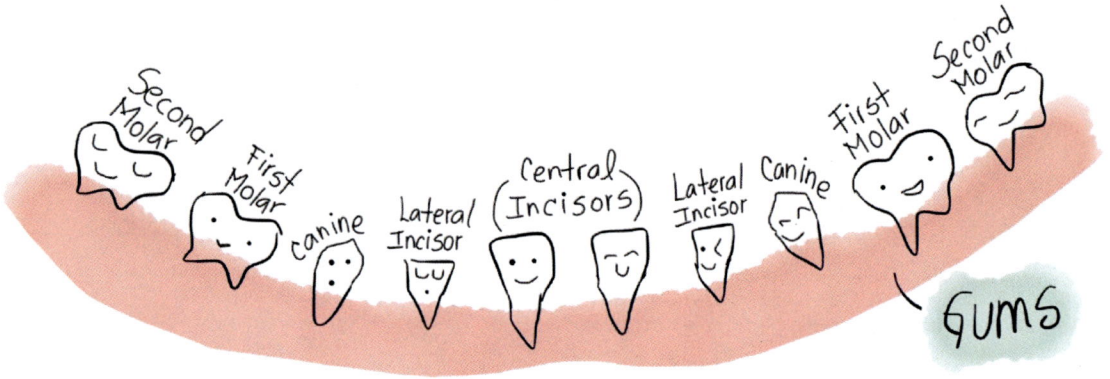

Second Molar
First Molar
Canine
Lateral Incisor
Central (Incisors)
Lateral Incisor
Canine
First Molar
Second Molar

Gums

Draw here

First, let's meet the tooth!

Parts of your tooth

CROWN

The part of your teeth that you can see in your mouth.

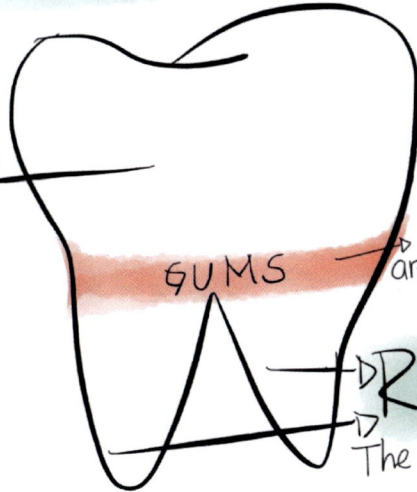

GUMS

All the pink gummy areas surrounding your teeth.

ROOTS

The part of your teeth that are inside your gums and bone.

Draw here

Now that you know the parts of your tooth, let's go to step 1!

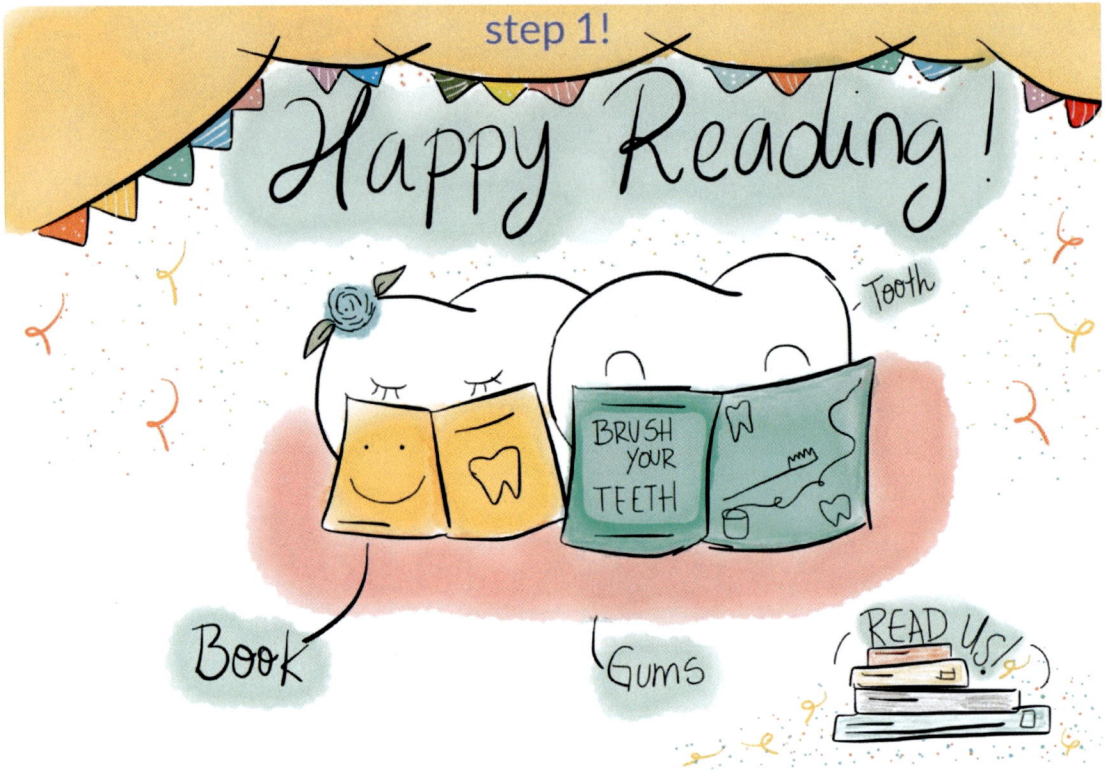

Happy Reading!

Tooth

BRUSH YOUR TEETH

Book

Gums

READ US!

Draw here

STEP 1
Eat in MODERATION whatever you want...

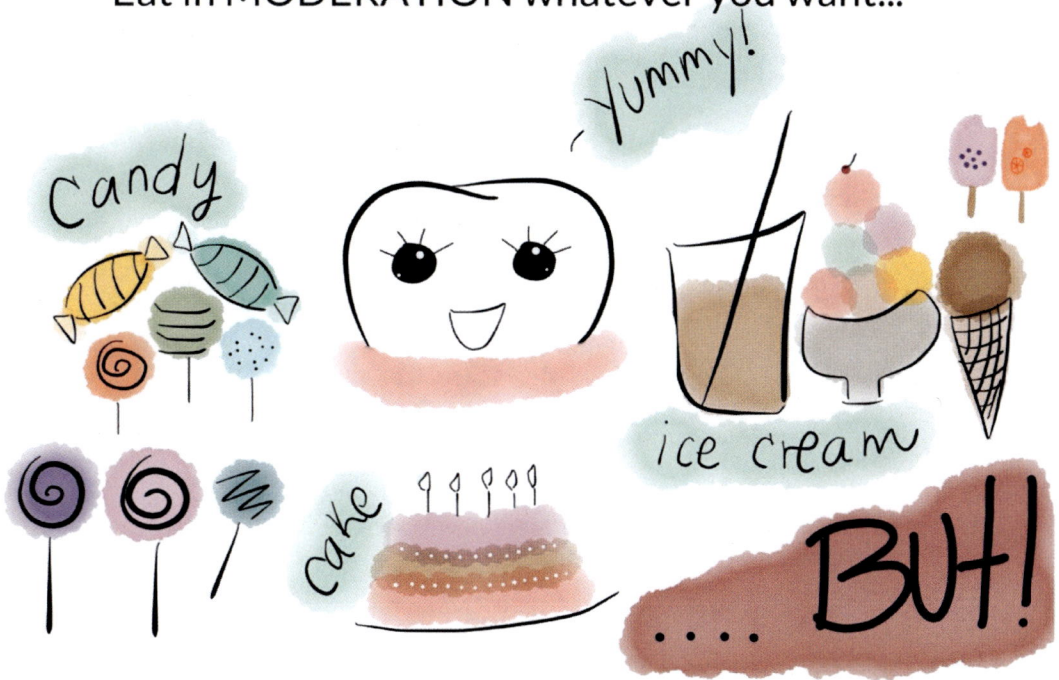

Yummy!

Candy

ice cream

cake

..... BUt!

Draw here

ALWAYS brush your teeth after every meal! I am sure you hear that almost every day, don't you?

ALWAYS

Woo-hoo! We are getting a shower!

Toothbrush

I am so happy!

Leftover candy

Toothpaste

RUN! Bacteria! RUN!

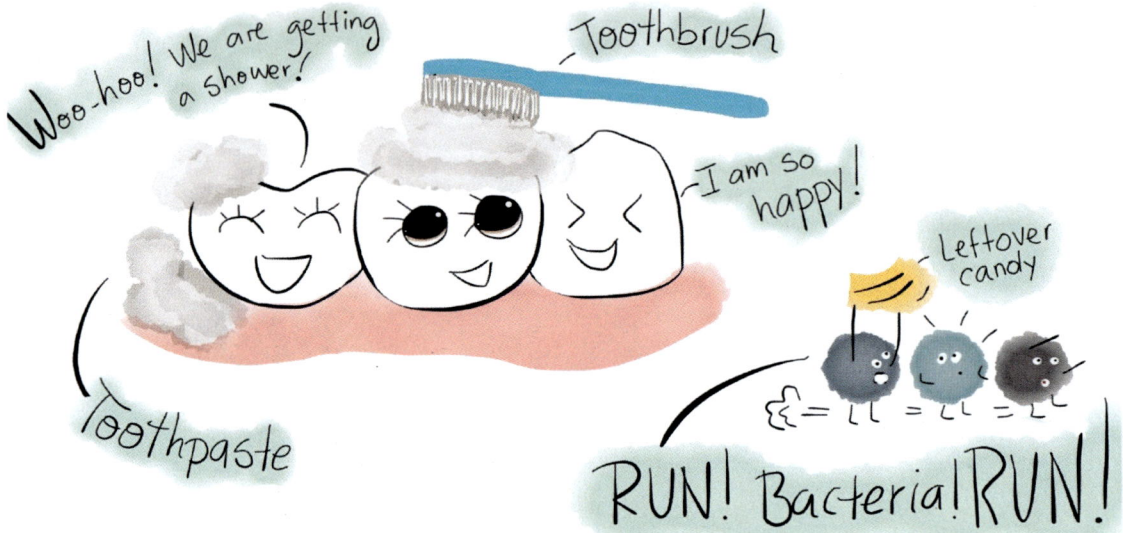

Let's go to the next page to find the answer!

Draw here

BACTERIA, the little bugs that you can see between both teeth in the drawing below. They start to accumulate more and more if we don't brush our teeth after eating. Bacteria live normally inside our mouths and they like candy too! like you! So, don't let them get out of control!

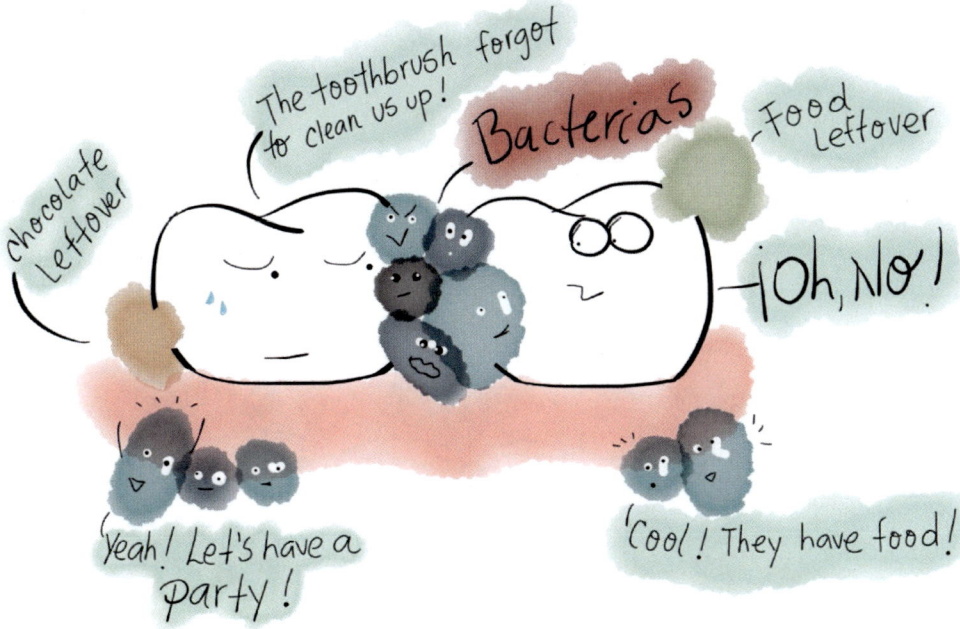

Draw here

These bugs (bacteria) get out of control, **if we don't brush our teeth.**

When they are out of control they start eating our teeth and making our gums sick!

More food!! Super!

The cake was good, man!

The best party!

The gums turn red and inflamed. Our teeth get black holes!(cavities) Cavities are those black dots that might appear on our teeth if we keep forgetting to brush our teeth.

So remember to brush your teeth every day to avoid bacteria creating a mess in your mouth.

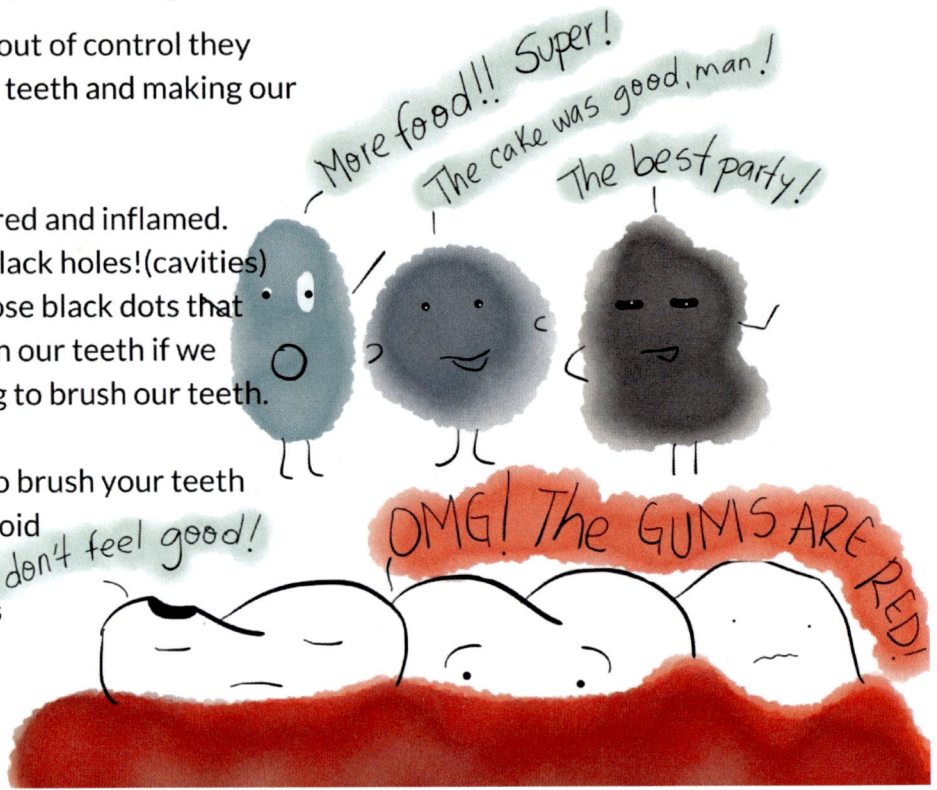

I don't feel good!

OMG! The GUMS ARE RED!

Draw here

Did you get it? I hope you did! So, now you know how to control bacteria

↓

BRUSHING YOUR TEETH AFTER EVERY MEAL! It is THAT EASY!

Do not let the gums turn red, inflamed. Do not allow your teeth to have cavities that can hurt a lot with time.

Look at your mouth in a mirror and tell mommy or daddy,
What do you see? Do you have black dots? Are your gums red or pink? What else do you see?

Draw here

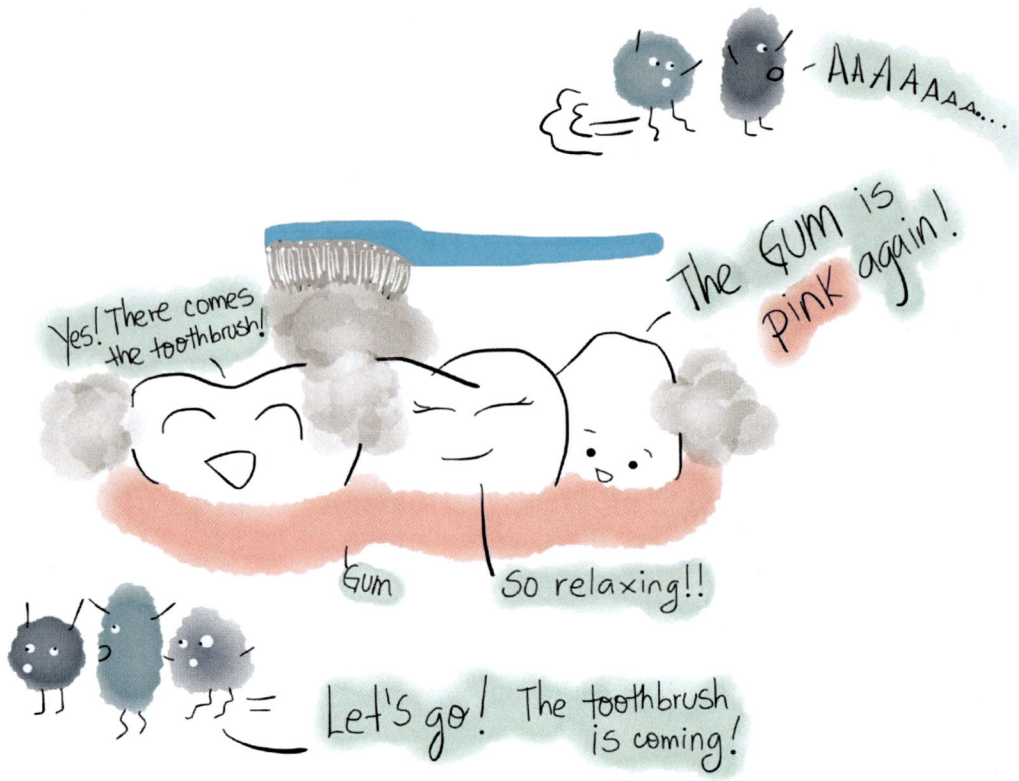

Draw here

STEP 2

REMEMBER! REMEMBER!

Brush all the surfaces of your teeth and use dental floss!

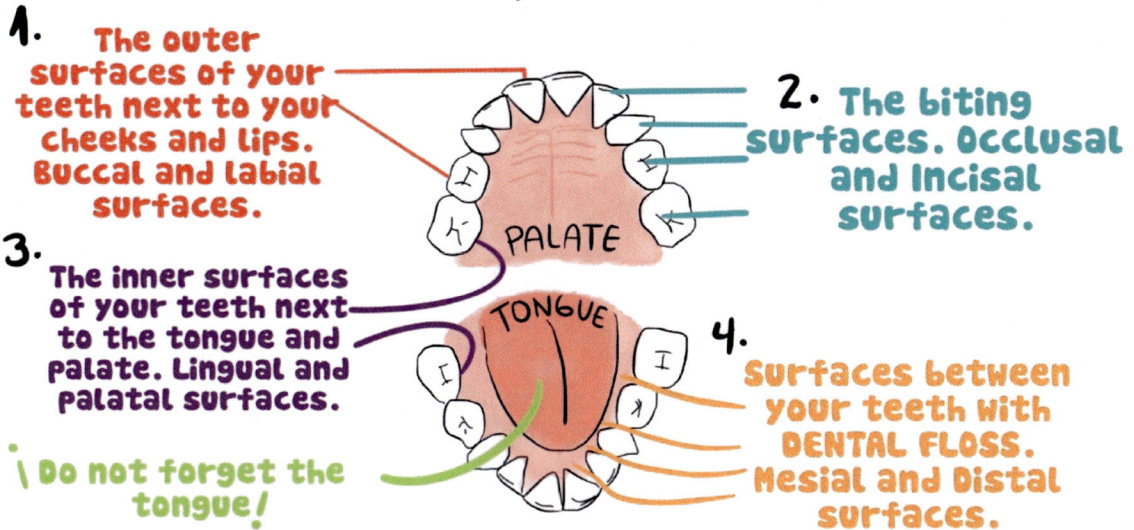

1. The outer surfaces of your teeth next to your cheeks and lips. Buccal and labial surfaces.

2. The biting surfaces. Occlusal and Incisal surfaces.

PALATE

3. The inner surfaces of your teeth next to the tongue and palate. Lingual and palatal surfaces.

TONGUE

4. Surfaces between your teeth with DENTAL FLOSS. Mesial and Distal surfaces.

Do not forget the tongue!

You can do circular-motion! Like if you were drawing a sun!(Circle). And up-and-down motion, like if you were brushing your hair. Easy to remember, right?

Draw here

STEP 3

Start using → dental floss. Ask mommy or daddy to help you. Use the tool known as flosser like the one in the image. Use it carefully or ask for help.

Dental Floss will always be the best option to clean **between** your teeth. That way you can have healthy gums and the surfaces between each tooth will be cavity free. Remember to do an up-and-down motion.

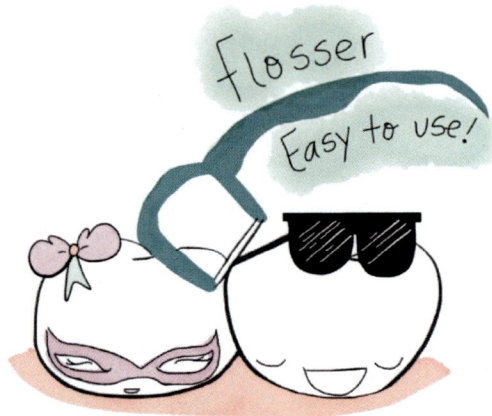

Flosser
Easy to use!

Draw here

Remember! Only the dental floss can enter between your teeth. (interdental spaces).
If you have crowded teeth, it is so important to ALWAYS use Floss. The leftover food and bacteria accumulate more due to the crowded position of your teeth. So, you will have to take special care of those specials spots.

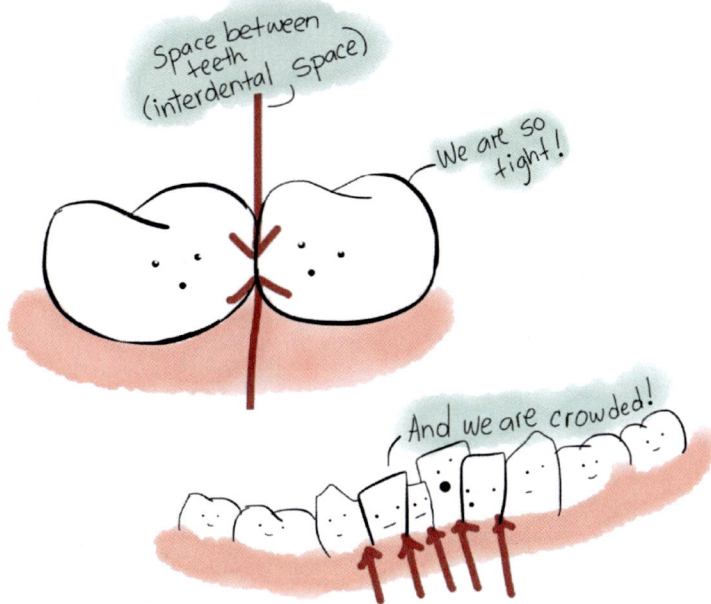

Draw here

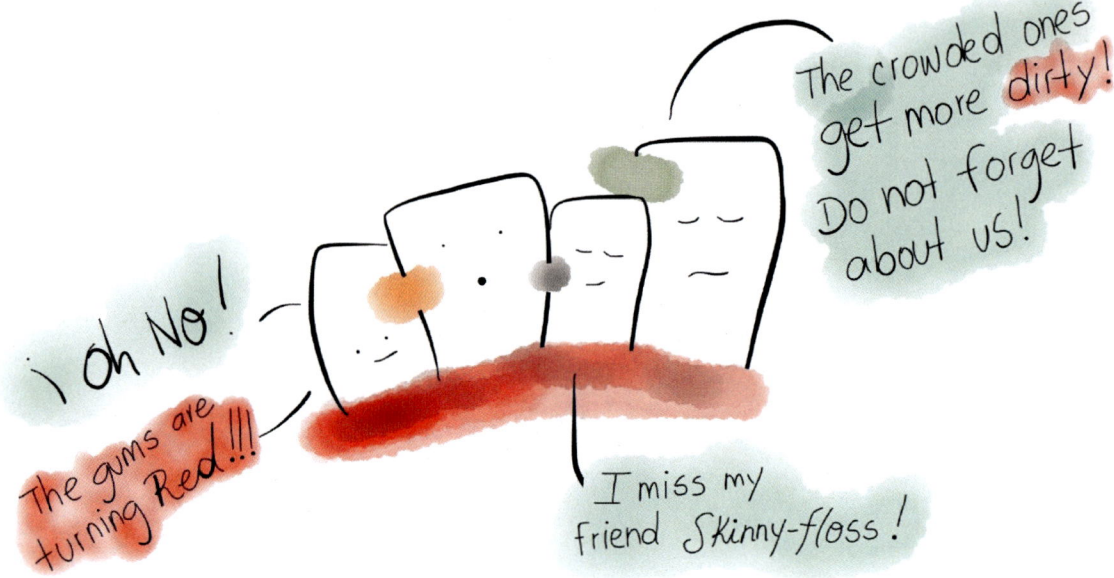

Draw here

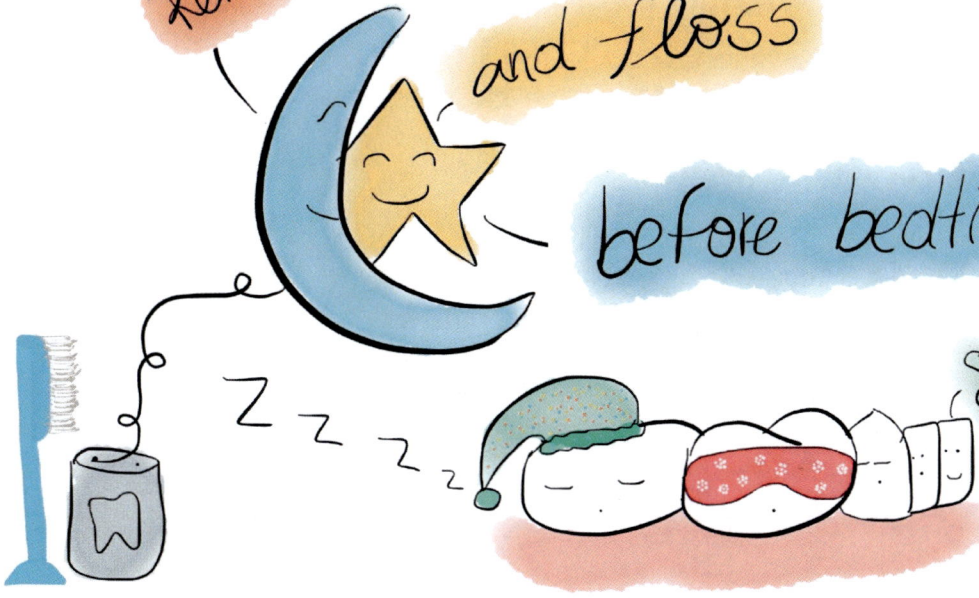

Draw here

STEP 4

Do not wait until you have a painful tooth to visit the dentist. If you allow this to happen it may be too late for the dentist to save your tooth. It is better to visit the tooth doctor every 3 to 6 months for a check-up to prevent sick teeth!

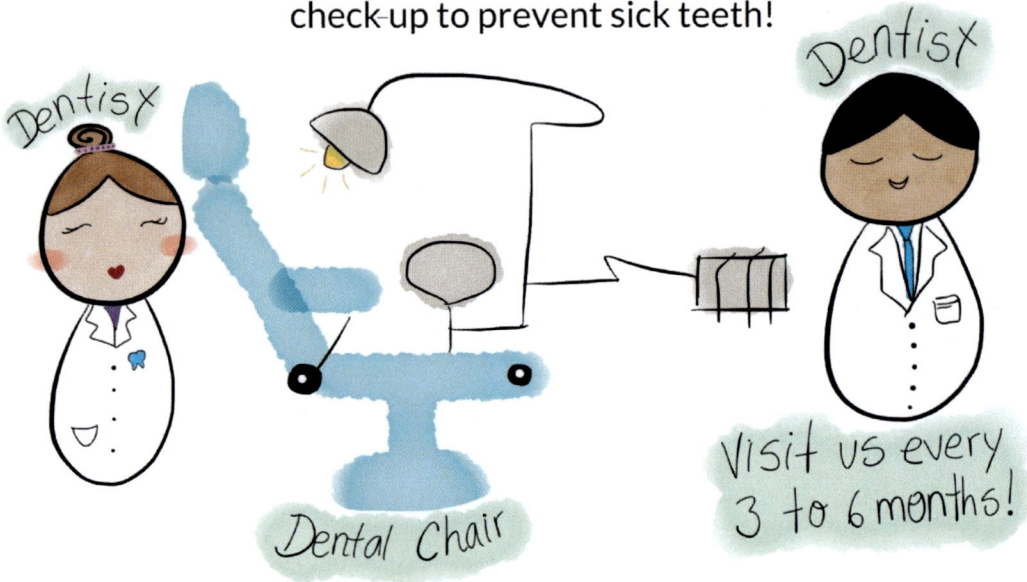

Dentist

Dentist

Dental Chair

Visit us every 3 to 6 months!

Draw here

Let's remember again!

Bacteria, out of control, cause:
-Cavities [black dots that could form into big holes (cavities)] in your teeth.

-Bad breath (who wants to have a smelly mouth? No one!

-And sick gums (red, bloody and inflamed gums).

All of the above is caused by bacteria out of control. Remember this happens because you didn't brush your teeth.
So, the nasty bugs (bacteria) grow out of control!

The Dentists are the only ones that can TREAT your sick teeth and gums! But do not wait until you go to the dentist to start taking care of your teeth! Only you can start taking care of your mouth from home! How? Tell mommy or daddy!
Now you know the answer!.

Draw here

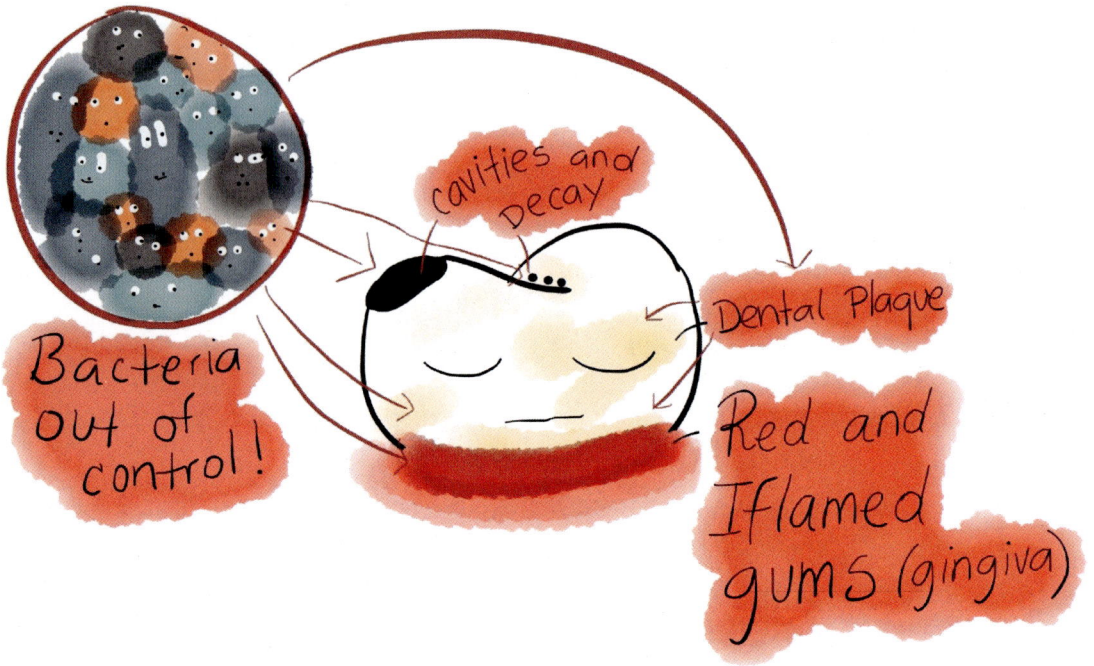

Bacteria
out of
control!

cavities and
Decay

Dental Plaque

Red and
Iflamed
gums (gingiva)

Draw here

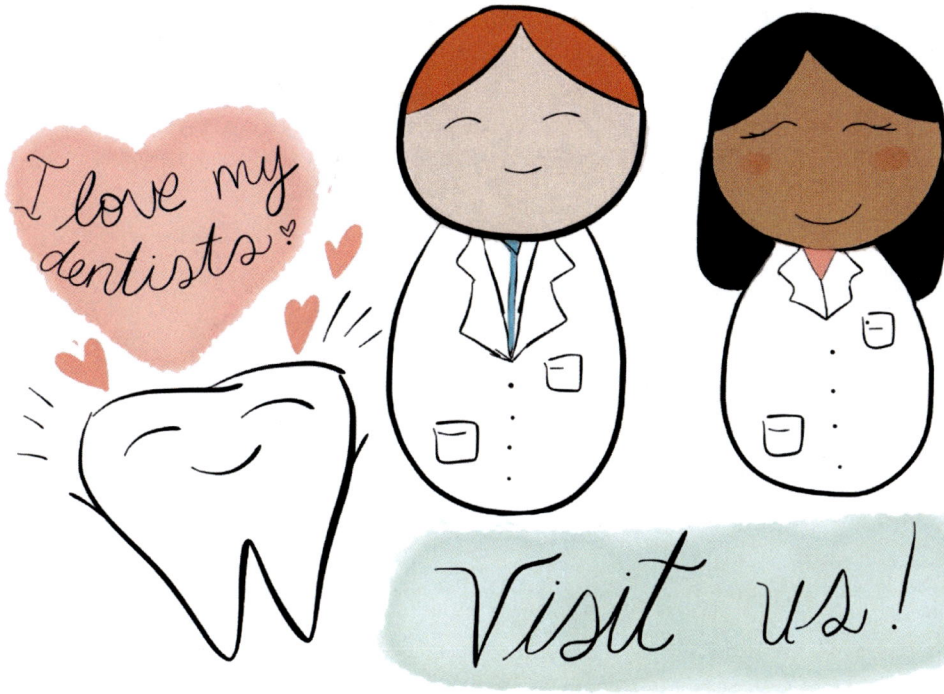
I love my dentists♥

Visit us!

Draw here

STEP 5

Very important! Wash your hands before eating, handling your toothbrush and after going to the bathroom! The germs can come into our body through our mouth! Let's wash our hands!

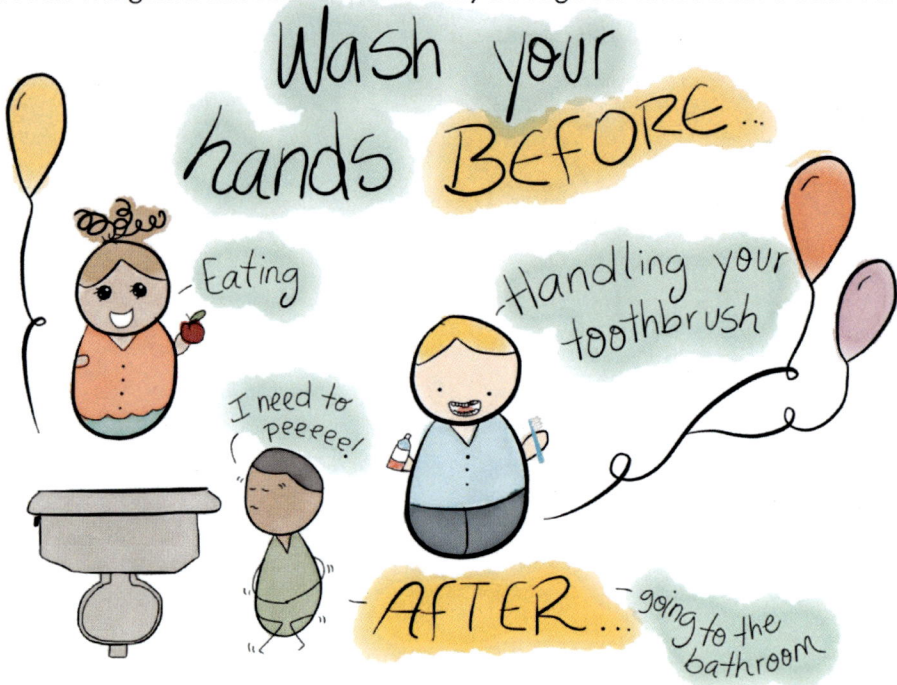

Wash your hands BEFORE...

- Eating

Handling your toothbrush

I need to peeeee!

- AFTER... - going to the bathroom

Draw here

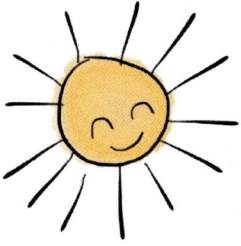
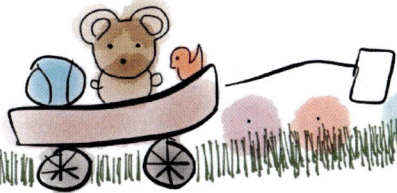

AFTER playing with your pets!

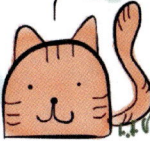
maya

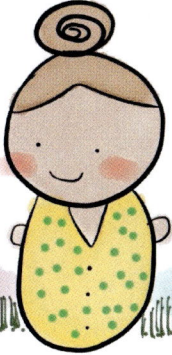

mimi

Draw here

Remember!

change your toothbrush

Every 3 MONTHs!

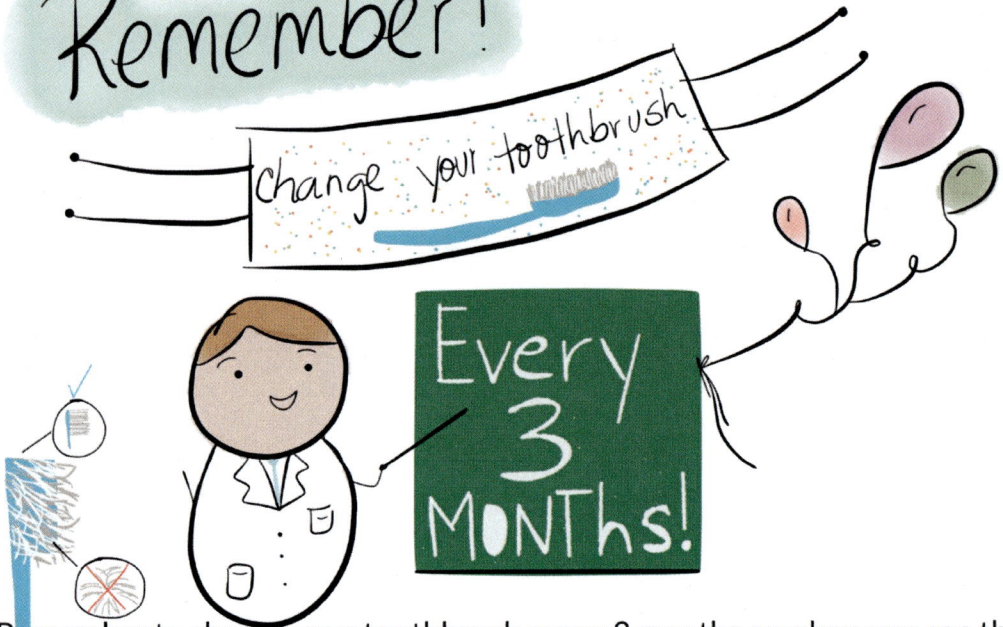

Remember to change your toothbrush every 3 months or when you see the bristles of your toothbrush starting to open out. Always place your toothbrush in a clean and dry area.

Draw here

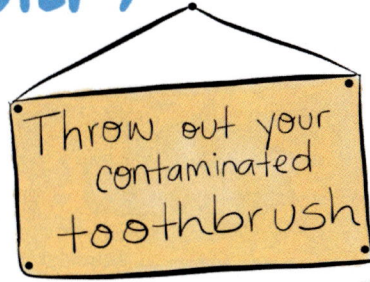

If you recently had the flu or if you
have been sick
with a gum infection,
change your toothbrush.
Why? Because you need to avoid
recontamination
with germs that are in
your toothbrush.
Do not put the old
dirty toothbrush in
your mouth.

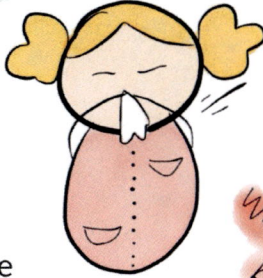

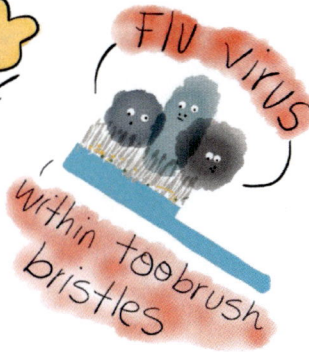

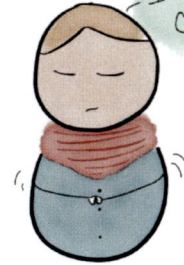

Because germs and
viruses stay within the
toothbrush bristles.
So, throw out your
contaminated toothbrush
and get a new one.

Draw here

Eat : Fruits and Vegetables of the season!

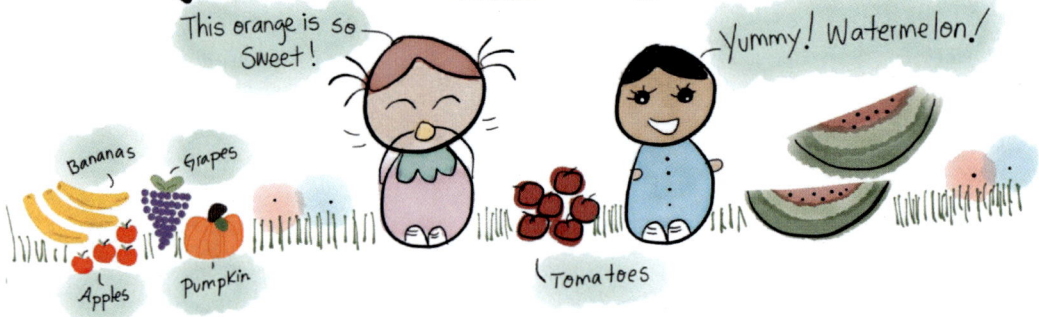

This orange is so sweet!

Yummy! Watermelon!

Bananas

Grapes

Apples

Pumpkin

Tomatoes

Eat fruits and vegetables! They have vitamins that help our body grow up healthy and strong and help fight back against diseases. Your teeth will be strong and healthy too! That is why it is very important to eat clean and healthy foods! Your body needs to be strong and a yummy way to achieve it, is to eat your favorites fruits and vegetables of the season!

Draw here

STEP 9

Help your little brother and sister to brush and use dental floss. You can share this information with your friends and help them too! That way more people will know how important is to take care of our teeth! Do not forget your pets! They have teeth too! Tell mommy or daddy to brush their teeth carefully or you can take them to the vet.

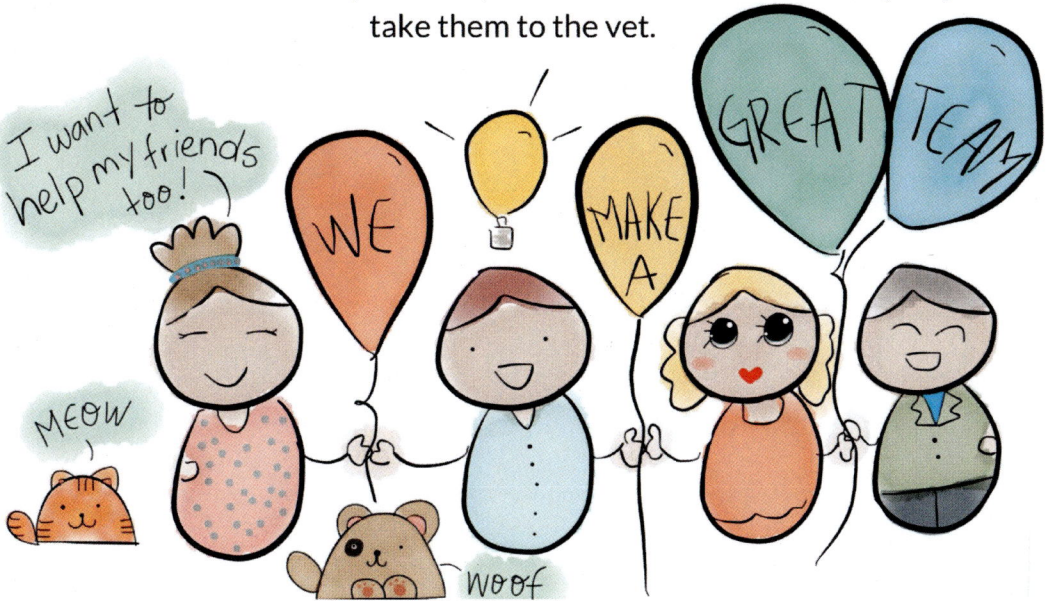

Draw here

STEP 10

Smile, Be Happy and Never Stop Dreaming! Never lose the motivation of taking care of your teeth! Remember that your mouth and teeth help you speak, eat and smile!. Be grateful for having them. Remember to always smile! Let's make a smiley world!

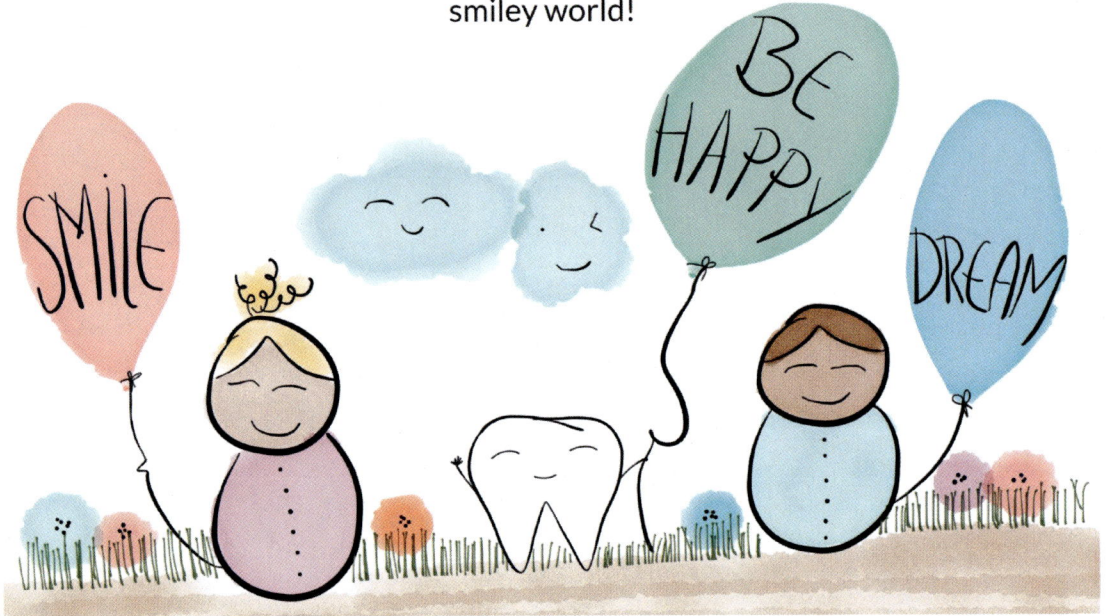

Draw here

Thank you
for
buying my guide!

Do you want to know more about your teeth? You can read my other book: How do I brush my teeth? available on amazon.com

You can find me on Instagram and Facebook as Happimola.

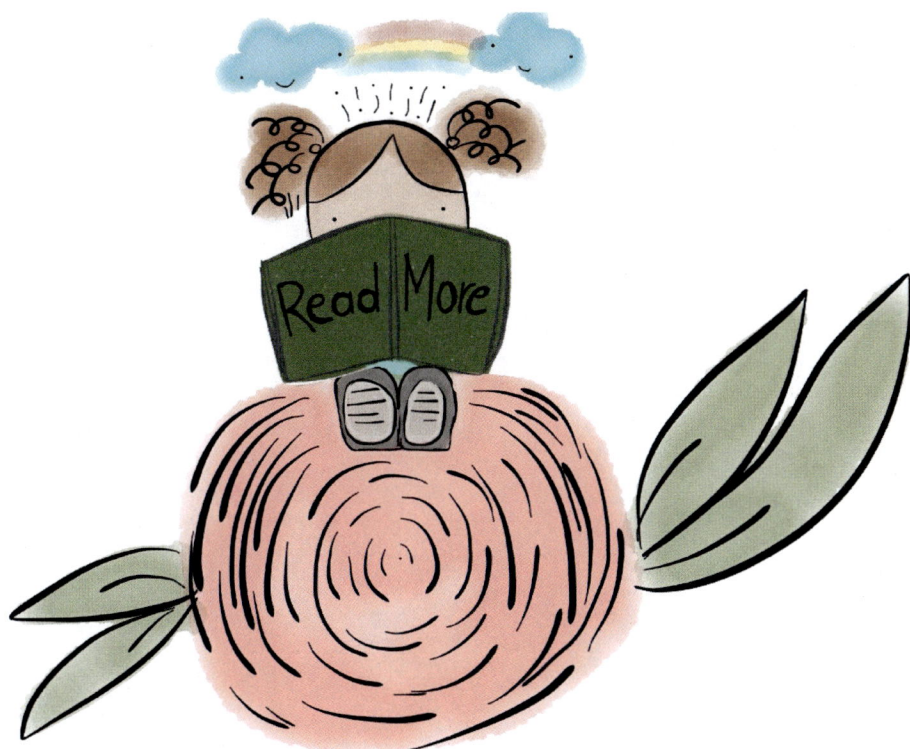

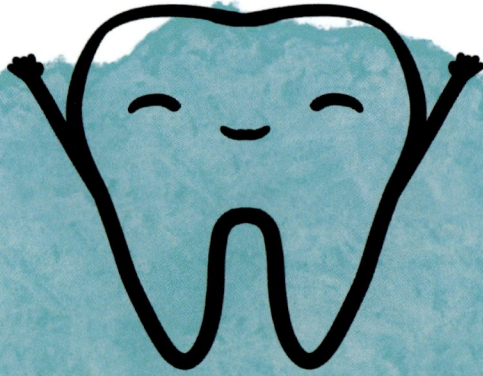

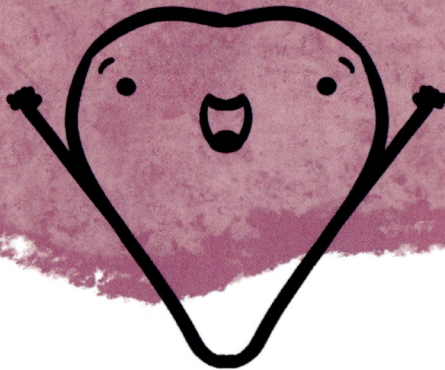

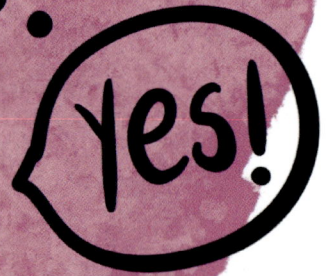

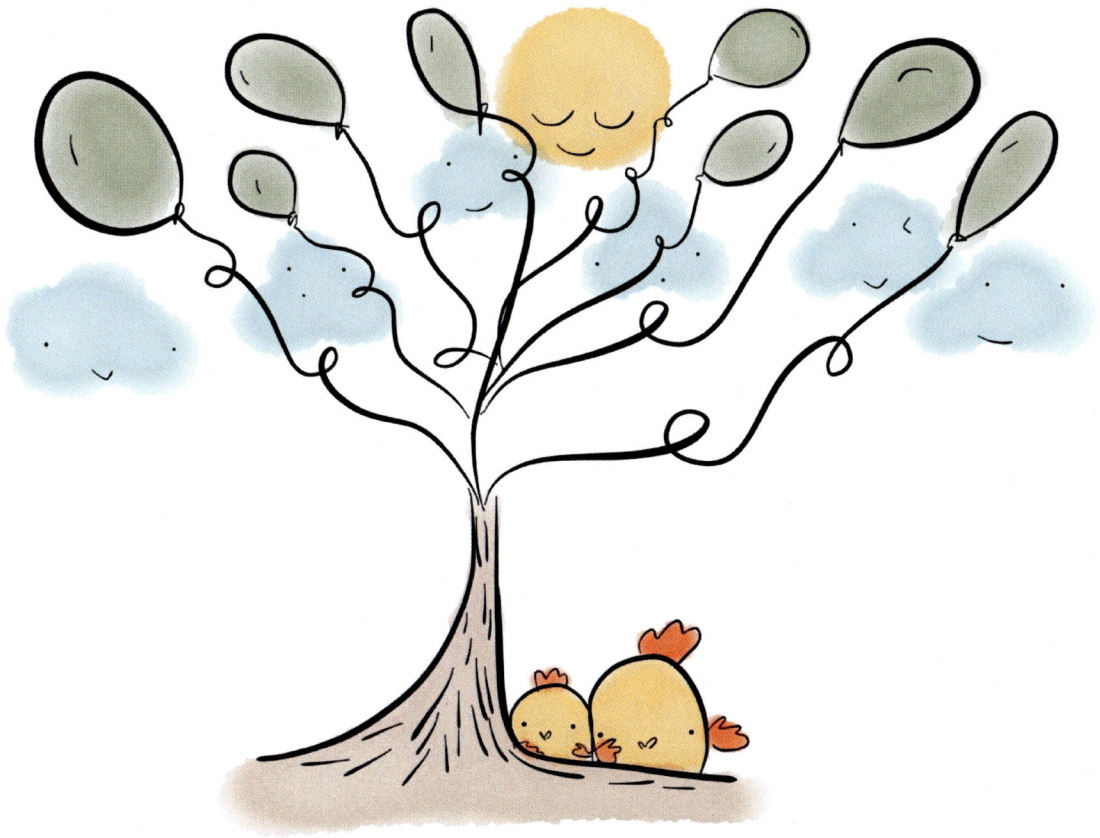

Imagine Your World With →

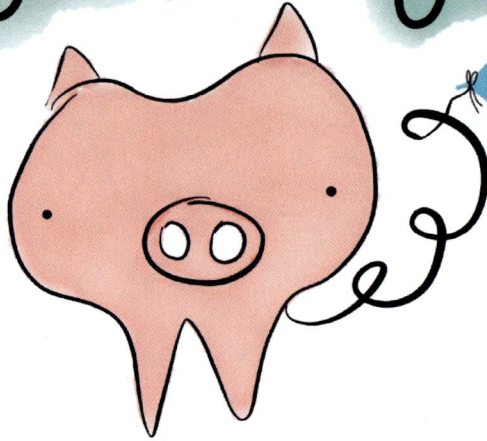

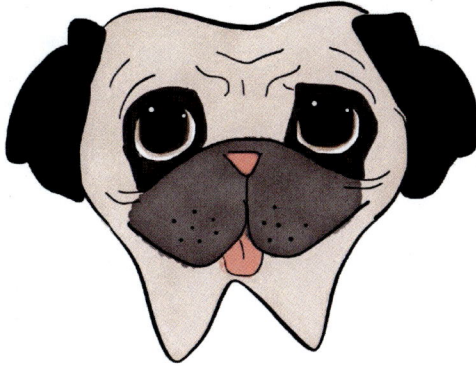

Molar Pug

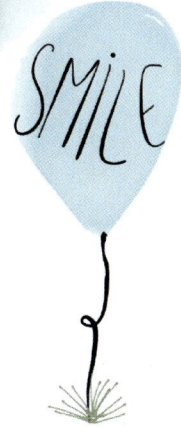

SMILE

Molar Cat

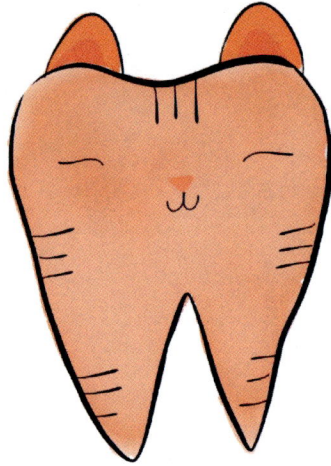

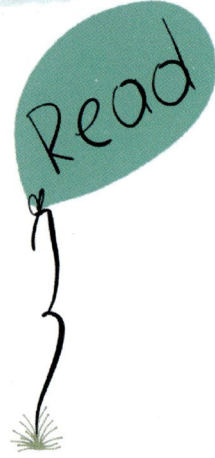

Read

Koala Baby Tooth

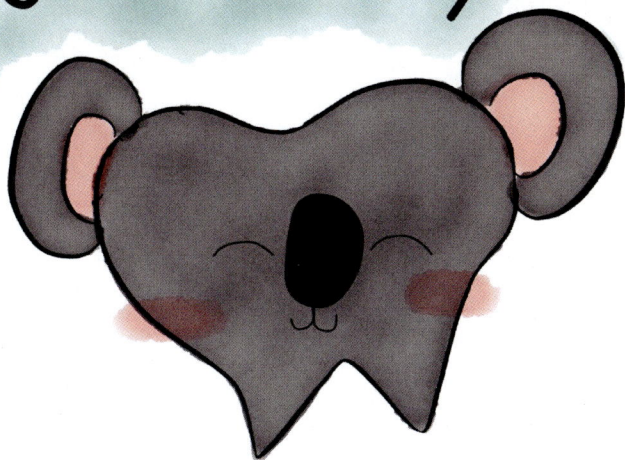

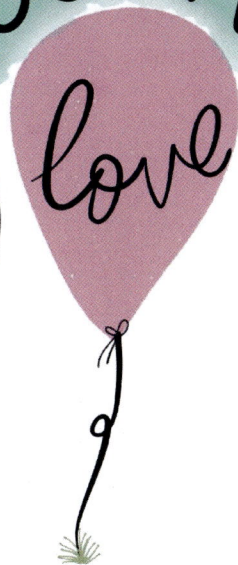

love

Molar Giraffe

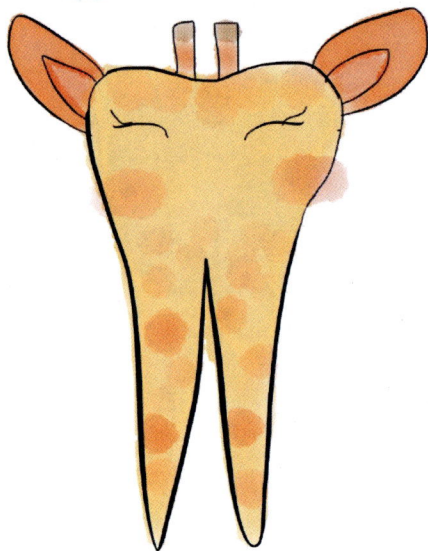

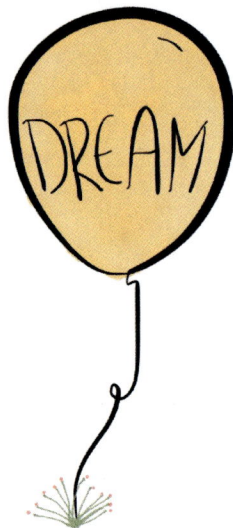

DREAM

Create Molar Robot

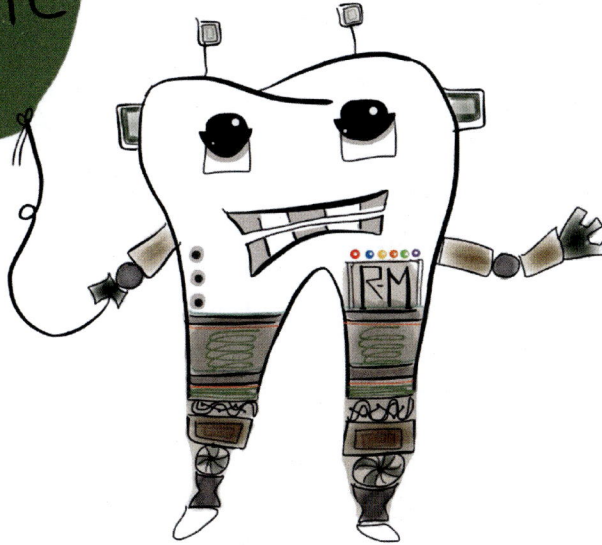

That
Would be
a funny
And
Extraordinary
World!

TAKE
CARE!

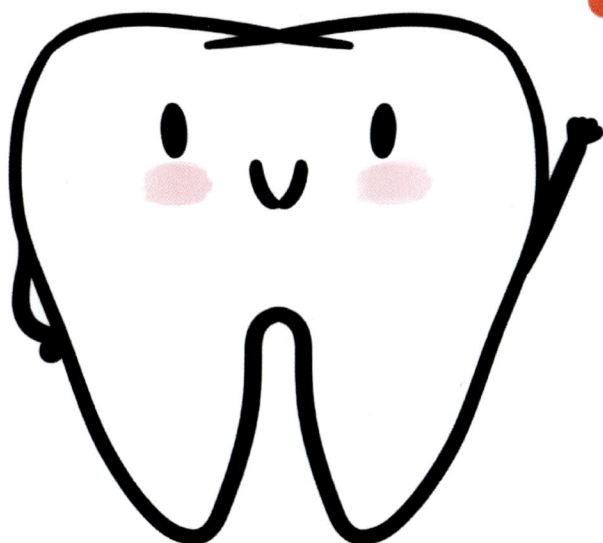

Made in the USA
Las Vegas, NV
02 June 2022

49652617R00026